CARNIVORE DIET

Get Strong and Ripped
With the Most natural Diet Ever-Burn Fat,
Build Muscle and Boost Strenght Easily
(Recipes Included)

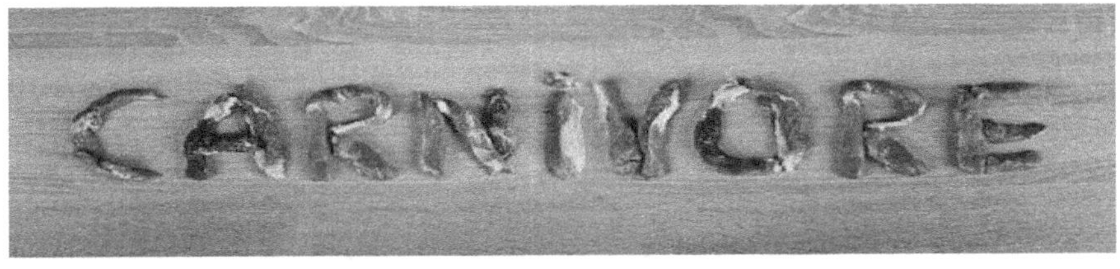

Table of Contents

Introduction

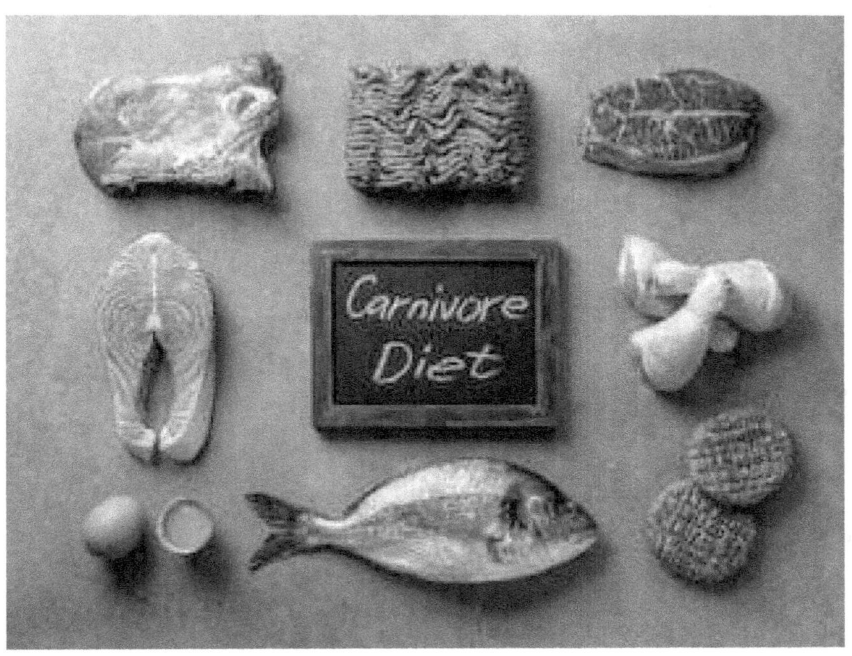

Over the years, men have evolved from one eating habit to the other due to varying factors and circumstances. As humans evolve and move from place to place, their eating habits also grow to meet current conditions. For some persons, a change in eating habits results from the desire to try new diet patterns; for others, the change might be triggered by one health condition or the other; or the quest to attain new health and/or physique status. Whatever the case may be, meals are eaten because of what they have to offer especially as it concerns nutritional benefits.

There are many meals named as superfoods and power diets due to their seeming nutritional benefits. Some of the purported health and dietary benefits have good scientific backups, while some are mere speculations with controversial scientific basis.

The focus has shifted from the foods that really matter and the result of this is the lot of health challenges we face in current times. Most times, the foods we embrace and cling so dearly to, are the ones with hazardous health challenges.

In the next few chapters of this book, we will be taking a trip through history, biology, and nutrition to find out what we are doing wrong as regards our diet, what we should and shouldn't eat, as well as some health changes we should make.

In this book, you will be introduced to the carnivore diet and be enlightened on how to make the best animal-based meals. You would then understand why *reading this book* might be your best shot at attaining perfect health and well-being.

Chapter One:
An Overview

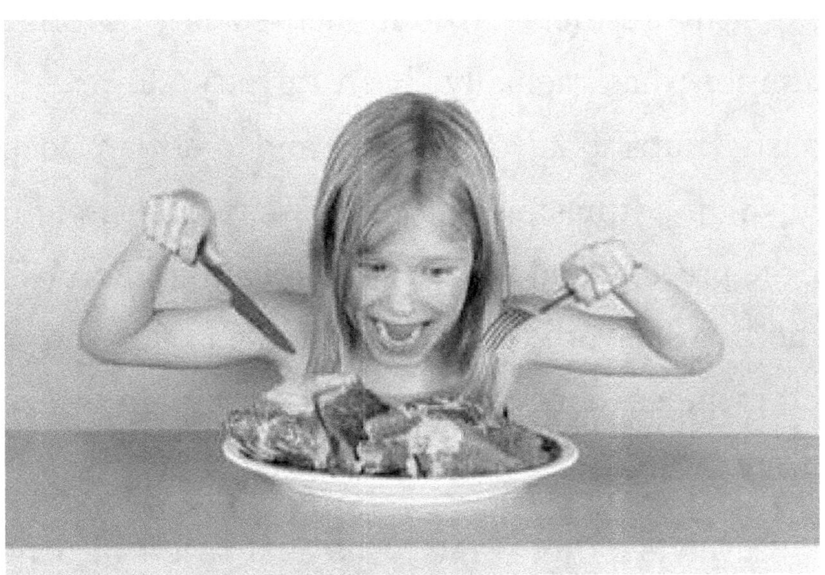

'Carnivore Diet' is a term used to represent a kind of diet that is strictly made up of meat, fish, and other animal foods, hence the name Carnivore. The Carnivore diet is hinged on eating only food from animal sources and excluding other foods such as vegetables, grains, fruits, nuts and the likes. It is also known as the Zero-carb diet but as many other diets increasingly pop up in recent times, it is safe to keep it at Carnivore diet.

As attempts to adequately and appropriately define the Carnivore diet has continued so far, no official definition has actually been given. However, a Holistic nutritional consultant and dietitian coach- Kelly Schmidt has a pretty impressive interpretation for the practice and it basically sums it up. According to her, a carnivore diet can be thought of as the diet that includes only foods that have either 'walked, flew, or swam.'

The Carnivore Diet came to be as a result of beliefs and researches that go back into time to trace the history of meals eaten by the human ancestral population and discovering it to be mainly made of meat and animal-based foods. These studies have also proposed that the deviation from the kinds of meals eaten in the historical part and the inclination towards high-carb meals is the major cause of many ailments and diseases we suffer today.

Just as every practice, theory, and belief stems from a source, Carnivore Diet also has its roots in the thoughts and beliefs and opinions of a particular person, after whom many came.

Former American orthopedic surgeon and author of the famous book 'The Carnivore Diet'- Shawn Baker is widely recognized as an advocate and a major leader of the Carnivore Diet movement. While proposing this diet, he cited proof of the effectiveness of the diet in treating and correcting various illnesses including diabetes, obesity, arthritis, depression, and many other diseases as he had noticed among a few persons who had been on the diet.

Engaging in the Carnivore diet in simple terms is ditching the diets high in carbohydrate and going after high protein, low carb, as well as quite a large amount of fat and healthy oil which is found in the carnivore diet. Many persons have referred to the practice as a pretty extreme one and it actually is; just as vegans cut out everything from their diet except plant-based food, Carnivores cut out everything except animal-based foods; two extremes, different points of focus. And while sticking to a carnivore diet might be extreme or difficult, with dedication and the drive to pursue it, it becomes a freeway to very healthy living.

To some, any meal plan that is not based on a balanced diet is not worth trying "so why then would I want to cut off grains and vegetables and stick to just meat?" You might ask. What if I tell you that all of the healthy nutrients you need to be healthy and fit are found in animal-based foods? Well, much later in the book the argument would make a lot more sense, and you might begin to see reasons why many have chosen to become Carnivores without as much as a second thought.

Taking a quick trip back to history, since about three million years ago man has been eating meat, and arguably more of meats than any other food products. There was never a time or period where meat was never a part of our diets as humans, and this goes to show that meat is the baseline food for man; it has been over time and would continue to be, regardless of reports that claim meats are responsible for heart diseases, cancer, and the likes. Interestingly, there have been verifiable claims that animal-based foods cure most of these diseases they are said to be responsible for.

For the sake of reference and mention as we go further in this book, a person or persons who practice the carnivore diet is referred to as a carnivore or carnivores and they are of different kinds, follow the diet for different reasons and also reap different benefits from the diet in the end.

Let us move on to identify the foods that can be eaten as part of the Carnivore diet and those that cannot.

Chapter Two:
Foods to eat; Foods to avoid

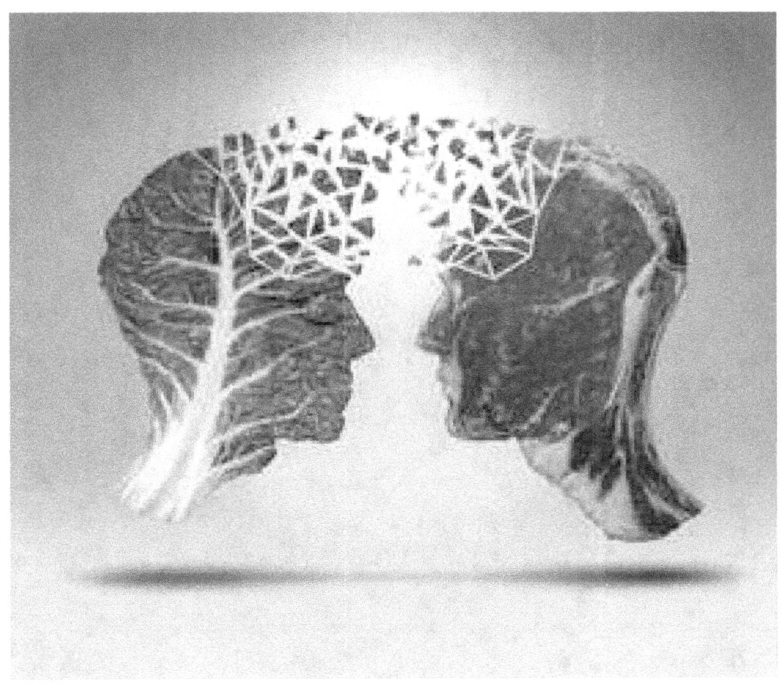

Just as we stated earlier, the Carnivore diet cuts out plant-based foods including grains, nuts and the likes and leaves us with lots and lots of meat, fish, egg, pork and the likes, as well as small amounts of dairy products that are low in lactose.

Now, let's have it in white and black- what goes and what does not when it comes to a carnivore diet; it is essential to draw the line so you can follow through correctly and avoid messing up your diet with avoidable mistakes. So, here is a list of the Dos.

Foods to Eat as part of the Carnivore Diet

- Beef

- Chicken

- Turkey

- White Fish

- Salmon

- Eggs

- Organ meats

- Pork

- Lamb

- Sardines

- Lard

- Bone marrow

- Poultry

- Bone Broth

- Salt and pepper

- Heavy cream (in small amounts)

- Hard Cheese (in small amounts)

All of the foods listed above are components of the Carnivores diet and can be eaten in whatever quantity as you desire asides for heavy cream and hard cheese that are specifically supposed to be taken in small amounts.

The Carnivore diet does not shy away from fatty meat; it is even advisably emphasized that the Carnivore eats the fatty parts of meat as they help to make up the daily energy requirements.

With regards to drinks: Tea, Coffee, and other plant-based drinks are discouraged but in their stead, lots of water and bone broth are more advisable. However, some Carnivores actually choose to leave tea and coffee as part of their diet (I mentioned ab initio that there are different types of carnivores).

You know what they say about gray areas and how things are not always black and white? Well, there are also some meals that may be acceptable as part of the Carnivore diet on the grounds that they actually come from animals. They include Cheese, Milk, and Yoghurt. The leader of the Carnivore diet Movement had earlier pointed out that these foods can be included based on their original sources; regardless, personal choice and decision will play a major role here in deciding whether or not you want them included as a part of your diet.

Foods that are not allowed as part of the Carnivore Diet

- Grains

- Legumes

- Vegetables

- Bread

- Seeds

- Pasta

- Nuts

- Fruits

- Snacks

- Baked foods

- Sugar

- Beverages

- Legumes

- Alcohol

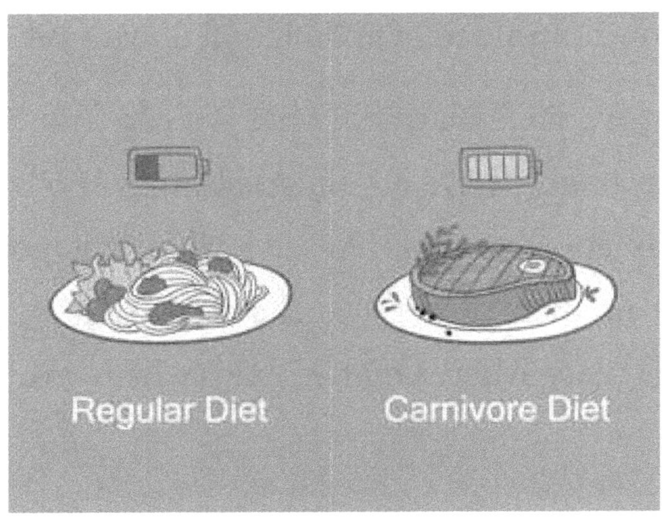

Basically, anything that is not meat or Animal-based is not allowed to be a part of your diet. We will go into recipes much later so you know just how much you can get out of the few foods you are allowed to consume, and believe me, you can do a lot.

No snacking before bed; no checking for calories when you eat, no worrying about how much weight you must have gained by eating your very favorite meal and what you have to do to work it off. The Carnivore diet is like an all-round solution to many worries and problems; you cut them off all at once and then look forward to living without these meals.

It is pretty daunting, I agree, but it is also pretty exciting and highly beneficial to your health: you just don't know how much of good it will do you yet.

Now that we have clarified what we can and cannot eat, you probably have an understanding of what this journey is going to look like and what it is going to take. Let us then proceed to the steps that will take you to the place where you become a carnivore

Chapter Three:
Steps to Becoming a Carnivore: Starting up on your Diet

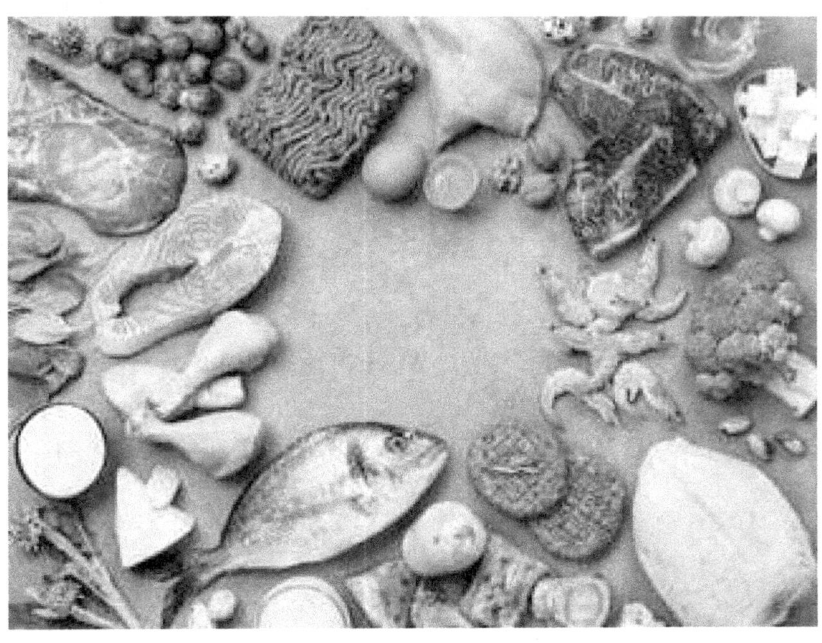

I have eaten whatever I wanted all my life, so where do I start? Simple! You just do. I will be a bit cliché and say 'leave the past behind and look ahead.' But truly, it is not the least bit easy, and it will even be more difficult for some people especially at the beginning. So here is a little something to guide you through the starting process

I. Start by cutting off beverages and Junk foods from your diet: Beverages and Soda can be pretty addictive- yes, I know that. In the same vein, they are practically the most unnecessary and equally harmful things you take into your body so let's start from there. Sodas and energy drinks add a very high amount of calories to your body and trust me, you don't want that! So as I see it, liquid calories gotten through sodas and beverages are the most unnecessary parts of your diet and you should eliminate them first.

Snacks are the next things you should absolutely eliminate from your diet; yes, you will be losing a lot of sweet stuff that you probably think you cannot do without, but in the real sense you can totally do without them. These junk foods we have come to love are doing more harm than good as they contribute lots of sugar, trans-fats, oils and sweeteners that you do not need. Trust me; cutting it off is best for you, even if you are not going the Carnivore way. Why would you then choose to keep stuffing yourself with foods that do absolutely nothing for you except for sweet taste?

First things first; cut off your intake of liquid calories and snacks and you're ready for the next step to living healthy on the Carnivore diet.

II. Get the Grains and Legumes off your daily menu: Now that you've done away with the most unnecessary and unbeneficial foods, it is time to get to the somewhat harder part especially as this might be where your all-time favorite meal falls into. Rice, Beans, Corn, Maize, Wheat, lentils, oats, and the likes are the foods we are talking about here.

Let me start by telling you that these meals are not as great as you think they are. First of all, they are not exactly great in nutritional composition, and when they do, your body is not able to absorb and digest them properly. Most of these foods also offer less nutritional benefits than Animal-based foods, so why hold onto something that would probably get stuck somewhere in your body and not do even the little it is supposed to?

Understandably, it might be challenging to remove all of these meals from your diet because they make up the major part of your daily meals, and you probably eat these meals at least once a day. Regardless, they have to go. Start it slowly and be determined to cut every one of them off.

III. Start monitoring your daily carb intake: Here's the deal; the Carnivore diet is Zero calorie, so once you start on the diet, you are going to cut off the intake of calories. For this exercise, the goal is to start cutting down macronutrients like carbohydrates, fats and proteins.

For your daily calorie intake, let's start by cutting it down to 100g per day. And yes, you're probably already yelling 'impossible' but it is not at all. The major reason you feel it is too high is because you are currently eating way above the regular healthy calorie intake.

While you are going to be cutting off major high carb meals, you can still stick to some foods that are below the 100 grams mark such as potatoes, low carb vegetables like spinach and broccoli, as well as fruits.

You are bound to feel the effect in the first few days and you might feel weak and tired, but it would get better and your body would eventually adapt and get used to it in no time.

IV. Start eating under 25 grams of carbs daily

I can imagine what is going through your mind right now, and yes, it gets worse, or better if you ask me. Once you have been able to start surviving eating under 100 grams of carbs daily and your body has adapted to it, it is time to cut closer and reduce your carb intake even more- we are heading to zero carbs after all.

This is the biggest stage after cutting down to 100g and most people face their greatest challenges here: some even fall off the wagon but if you have gone so far, then you should take it all the way.

You are going to have to restrict your meals mainly to low carb vegetables and move away from most of the meals you ate when sticking to the 100g diet. It is hard, it is very hard, but is it worth it? Totally!

V. One more thing, Oils and vegetables!

This should be easy, right? We shall see about that.

Vegetables and oils are the next things to go down from your diet just before you are all set to become a carnivore. Remember we are going Animal-based and vegetables and edible oils don't fall in this category. So we take them out.

Vegetable oils are not always good for you; sometimes they actually do you more harm than good especially when fried or heated. You might have to let go of all kinds of vegetable except olive oil which you can continue using at your own discretion albeit in small amounts.

Vegetables have to go too. I know you think they are really healthy, helps you grow stronger and all of that but you truly don't need vegetables and you can definitely do without them. So it is goodbye to spinach, cucumbers and lettuce and all of the veggies and welcome to meat.

VI. Animal- based foods only

In case there is anything we haven't mentioned, well, is it animal based? No? Then it goes out too.

At this point we are totally avoiding anything that is not animal based and sticking to animal products only; at this point you can call yourself a carnivore.

Now you will only eat things gotten from animals: Meat, fish, chicken, pork, lamb, eggs and the likes. Like I mentioned earlier, some persons include little amounts of milk and cheese as well, but some don't' this is where strictness in terms of diet comes in.

At this point, some carnivores will allow coffee, milk and cheese while others will choose to stay away from all of them. It is up to you to choose what your body would adapt to strict or easy. Regardless, these things should be added in very small amounts and scarcely as well so as not to mess up the whole progress.

As we move on, you will find out more and even ways to make your unique carnivore diet and enjoy it.

Chapter Four:
Benefits And Superpowers Of Carnivore Diet And Animal-Based Foods

NUTRITIONAL VALUE OF DIFFERENT ANIMAL BASED MEALS

Animal based Meals	Protein (g)	Total Fat (g)	Cholesterol (mg)	Calories	Iron (mg per 100g)	Saturated fat
Salmon Fish	25	14	71	233	1	2.8
White Fish	27.3	1.7	132	132	1	0.4
Pork (tenderloin, steak)	31.8	5.4	89	185	0.7	1.9
Pork (Ham, Roasted)	25.6	10.2	67	201	1	3.5

Chicken (Breast, no skin)	35.1	4.1	96	186	0.8	1.1
Lamb (Leg, roasted)	32	8.7	101	216	1.5	3.1
Lamb (Shank)	31.8	7.6	98	203	1.5	2.7
Bison	34.1	5.6	89	197	n/a	2.5
Ostrich	28	2.5	50	135	n/a	0.5
Kangaroo filet	22.1	1.3	56	103	2.6	0.3
Beef (Steak)	34.2	7.5	75	212	2.5	3
Beef (Extra lean gound)	29.2	6.7	86	185	2.5	

There are quite a number of benefits associated with the Carnivore diet including managing and curing diabetes, heart diseases as well as other major health issues. People who have tried the diet and currently live on the Carnivore diet have pointed out a couple of things that the diet has done for them. However, the benefits of the Carnivore diets vary according to who is dieting and who you ask.

Generally, improved energy, increased athletic prowess, weight loss, reduced gastrointestinal stress, reduction of sugar level, and weight reduction are a few of these benefits.

Meats boast of a lot of Vitamin B, especially B6 and B12. Vitamin B tends to improve the symptoms of lupus and vitamin B6 particularly has been linked to the correction of immune function in people with lupus as well as suppression of inflammation in these persons.

According to a Chinese study cited in the European Journal of Epidemiology, children who eat meat are more likely to have increased cognitive functions later in life when compared to children who do not. This goes to show a very large correlation between meat intake and improved cognitive function.

Many people who observe the Carnivore diet have often claimed to experience a form of mental clarity, reduction in brain fog, as well as a kind of mental and physical calm that was previously out of reach when they lived on carbohydrate diets.

Some Health Benefits Of The Carnivore Diet

The following benefits are reported by persons who have practiced the diet and reaped its benefits

1. Improved mood and energy

2. Reduction of inflammation and inflammatory diseases

3. Speedy recovery time

4. Improved athletic performance

5. Better skin conditions and cure of eczema

6. Quick weight loss among overweight people

7. Perfect appetite management and control

8. Reduced gastrointestinal problems

9. Reduced joint pain.

10. Testosterone health

Apart from the above-listed benefits, there have been personal testimonials from people who have lived on the diet for a while and experienced the benefits of this diet.

Personal Testimonials

Mikhalia Peterson: the daughter of lifestyle guru Jordan Peterson, her diet which constituted solely of beef, salt, and water actually provided relief for her depression. In the August 2018 edition of the times, she testified of the benefits of the diet to her health alongside her father.

Jordan Peterson: a clinical psychologist who practices the Carnivore diet. According to him, the diet has saved him from a lifelong fight with depression.

A former Vegan and mother of three has given accolades to the Carnivore diet as well as a bodybuilder who lost 210 pounds simply by taking on the carnivore diet and the pictures of these people are up on the social media handle of Carnivore diet advocate, Shawn Baker (who had introduced them to the diet).

I have also put together a list of claims and testimonials by different people who are currently Carnivores from different social media pages and platforms and these are a few of the Diseases they testify to have been cured by eating nothing but Animal-based foods.

- Diabetes

- Epilepsy

- Cancer

- Autism

- Heart Diseases

- Endometriosis

- Multiple sclerosis

- Arthritis

- Polycystic ovarian syndrome.

There are many other testimonials regarding different benefits of the Carnivore Diet by different persons and like I mentioned earlier, the benefits depend on who you ask.

Let's take a quick look at some biological arguments in favor of the Carnivore Diet

Arguments For The Carnivore Diet
Below are a few biological arguments in favor of the Carnivore Diet and Animal-based plants.

- Meat nutrients are majorly bioavailable: All the amino acids we need to live and thrive are found in meat. It is also easier to absorb these nutrients because they are in animal form, and do not need conversion to be absorbed; as opposed to plant nutrients that would need to go through some conversation processes. Some essential nutrients like vitamin B12, creatine, carnosine and the likes only exist naturally in meat, and this diet gives you full access to these nutrients. The best thing, therefore, is to obtain these nutrients the easier way from Meats.

- Meat is very safe compared to plants in terms of toxins: Plants contain many toxins that could be harmful to the person who eats it especially in form of pesticides, treatment and the likes but animals are mostly free of these toxins as they are able to fend for themselves while they are alive.

Chapter Five:
Effects of Carnivore Diets on Weight loss

If there is one thing the Carnivore diet has been appreciated for by people, it is for its major effect in smooth and healthy weight loss. Many people have testified about losing massive weight as a result of this diet and still remaining healthy during and after this process but let us take an in-depth look at the effects of animal-based diets on weight loss.

Some studies by The National Institutes of Health have shown that low carb and high protein diets actually help in weight loss. This is largely due to the fact that protein generally makes you feel full faster after eating very little; when you feel full early, you eat less thereby reducing your calorie intake and engineering weight loss. When you eat meat or other animal-based foods regularly, you are on the large scale eating less than you would when you are eating legumes, grains, vegetables and the rest that are high in carbs.

On a short term basis, the Carnivore diet can really work wonders when it comes to weight loss: reducing what you eat, satisfying you earlier and keeping you healthy.

A 2012 publication by the US library of Medicine National Institute of Health showed results of a 3 month study carried out on 132 adults suffering obesity and excessive weight. These adults were on 4 energy- restricted containing different amounts of carbs and proteins. Results of the study showed that persons who ate more high-protein diet lost considerably more fat and weight than those who ate lower protein and higher carb diets. You can see for yourself here the power of high protein diets.

Further studies by the National Institute of Health have also shown that reduction of carb intake goes a long way to more sustainable and long-lasting weight loss. Also, eating meals less in calories and high in protein is a widely acceptable weight loss choice.

According to Kelly Schmidt, the carnivore diet eliminates mindless eating and increases satiety, which automatically reduces your Calorie and overall intake. The fact that you are eating only one type of food reduces your calorie intake and gives you a more healthy protein. However, it is essential for you also not to overeat this protein in one fell swoop because too much of everything is bad, isn't it?

Many people have turned to the Carnivore Diet as it offers a very quick road to weight loss: quicker than many other forms of dieting. It works rapidly, and it has had a major impact on the lives of many people trying to combat weight gain. Regardless, losing excess weight is not the end of it; you also have to work hard to maintain your current weight.

The Carnivore Diet And Reduced Symptoms Of Autism

The National Institute of Health, there are quite a large number of nutrients present in meats and other proteins that reduce the symptoms of autisms. Cysteine, an amino acid that is present in meat at high levels, has been very closely linked to the reduction of symptoms of autism in patients. Nearly every component of the Carnivore Diet is higher in cysteine than other diets and so this is a good source of the vital nutrient.

Oily fish such as sardines and salmon are rich in omega 3 fatty acid which has also been linked to improvements in the symptoms of autism. Therefore, an increased intake of oily fish would go a long way to treat the symptoms of autism, and this is according to Neuropsychiatric Disease and treatment by Yu-Shian Cheng et al.

Zinc, according to Front Synaptic Neurosis (2018) by Simone Hagmeye and others, increases regulatory T cells and is beneficial to people with autoimmunity. Zinc supplements have been very beneficial for some persons suffering from autism, and with the abundance of Zinc in meat, there is a tendency to increase and improve symptoms of the disease in some people.

Chapter Six:
Squashing Myths regarding
Animal-based meals

- Meats are not good for you; they rot in your colon: Many people who oppose meat-eating have given flimsy claims to dissuade people; one of these claims is that meat rots in your colon.

First of all, who even says something like that? I really don't understand the reasoning behind it, but some people seem to believe it so let's squash it right now.

Like every other food, when we eat meat, it gets broken down by digestive enzymes. The proteins are broken down into amino acids in the small intestine while the fats are broken into fatty acids. After everything has been broken down, it gets absorbed into the bloodstream.

It is truly a wonder how people came about this theory but meat doesn't rot in the colon or anywhere else. You know what doesn't get broken down and rots in your stomach? It is fiber from fruits, vegetables, legumes and the likes that does not get broken down. This is because the digestive system cannot break down the fiber gotten from some of these foods, and they eventually get sent into the colon where they get rotten.

So you see, whoever said this had it all wrong.

• Meat Causes Type 2 diabetes and heart diseases

Meat has been continuously blamed for many diseases especially heart diseases and type2 diabetes, but you know the funny thing? These diseases that have been linked to meat consumption are relatively new to us so how could they have been caused by meat we have been eating since the existence of man?

Research shows that humans have been eating meat for millions of years, and there was never a mention of heart diseases among these people so something else has to be responsible for heart diseases and diabetes and it is definitely not meat.

Here is the squash for this assumption, and trust me; it is something that cannot be contended — a 2010 study 'Circulation. Author manuscript; available in PMC 2011 Jun 1' gathered data from about 20 studies which included 1,218,380 people. At the end of this research, there was no link proven between the intake of meat and heart diseases.

The only link that could be found was the link between the diseases and processed meat; which is definitely not something I would advise you to eat. It is important that you eat only healthy meat and healthy foods in general.

So you see, even this assumption is wrong.

- Meat is filled with Harmful Fat and Cholesterol

You must be wondering if I am going to counter this too; yes, I am.

We know that meat is high in cholesterol and fat, but the question is, is it harmful fat? No. cholesterol is an important molecule in the body, and it is present in every cell membrane.

You know how important cholesterol is? It is so important that even the liver produces cholesterol in addition to the one we take in. American Health Journal (1996) states that when we get lots of cholesterol from our meals the liver produces less to balance it up and when we eat less, the liver increases the amount of cholesterol it produces.

- Red Meat causes Cancer

It is a widespread fact that processed meat is associated with an increase in the risk of cancer and I am not about to discredit all the years of research that has been put into this one, but I am going to point out something that most people miss when quoting the results of such research.

A research by the international Association for the study of Obesity (2010) has shown that the effect of unprocessed red meat on women in relation to cancer is nonexistent, while among the men, it is extremely low. This brings us back to what I had earlier said about choosing fresh raw meat and making your meal rather than going after processed meats.

After choosing to get fresh meat, the method of cooking is also something to look out for because the way you cook your meat also has an effect on your body. When meat is overcooked, it can form some compounds that might be harmful to the body.

Don't get worried yet, I mean, every meal has its peculiarities and there are things to watch out for whether you are eating grains or vegetables so this is just one of such measures for meat. All you have to do is cook your meat carefully and look for gentler methods to cook your meat and at all costs, avoid eating it if it is burnt.

- Meat is unhealthy for your bones

There are beliefs that too much protein in the body increases the loss of calcium, thereby affecting the growth and development of bones among the young and old alike. But this is not exactly how these things work; here is what happens

As opposed to claims that protein leads to osteoporosis, the evidence of quite a number of researches shows that high protein consumption actually leads to improved bone density and invariably lowers the risk of osteoporosis. Research on dietary protein by the US Library of medicine has also correlated this claim.

- Meat is unnecessary; you can do without it

A lot of the nutrients found in meat is also found in other animal-based foods and that is a fact I would agree to; however, these nutrients are not found in foods that are not plant-based, so this does not mean that you can replace meat with oats or rice because they don't contain these nutrients. What you can do is to eat meat interchangeably with other animal-based foods but then isn't that what carnivores do?

Notwithstanding the claims that meat is unnecessary, there are nutrients found in meat and other animal-based foods that are very important; Take protein, creatine, carnosine, vitamin B6, B12, fat-soluble vitamins as a few of these nutrients.

There is meat, and there is quality meat; quality meat is the perfect diet because it boasts of so many nutrients: even those that have not been discovered.

Vegans say that you can do without meat, and you actually can. The question is, do you want to live without meat, and why would you want to do that? We can survive without many groups of food but it doesn't mean we should choose to survive without them and meat is one food you should not choose to live without.

- Humans are naturally Herbivores

I mean, why do we still have these back and forth arguments, especially with the vegans who believe that human ancestors ate plants and not meat. Well, our research has proven otherwise and we can say on authority that our ancestors have been eating meat for millions of years and the human body is very much adapted to the consumption of meat.

Taking a look at our digestive system can convince you that our body is made for eating and digesting meats and other animal-based foods. Enzymes and acids in the body are very much present to break down these proteins so why would anyone say we were not meant to eat meat? We have systems in place for the digestion of these foods which invariably means we can eat them and we definitely should eat them.

Some brain studies I quote earlier also showed that the consumption of animal foods which obviously include meat is linked to the evolution and development of the brain especially among youngsters.

• Meat makes You Fat

Many people say 'don't eat meat, you will get fat' and when you ask them the reason for their statement they say it is because red meat contains a lot of fat. But here is something you should know: Meat is very rich in bioavailable protein which is very instrumental in weight loss.

Rather than cutting off meat and eating other food when you are trying to lose weight, the best thing to do is actually to cut off other foods and focus on only meat.

A study featured in the American Journal of Clinical nutrition (2005) has found that when you increase the amount of protein in a diet, you automatically cut down the calorie intake which automatically leads to weight loss.

Another reason why it doesn't make sense for meat and animal-based foods to make you fat is that the more protein you eat tends to increase your muscle mass.

Chapter Seven:
Testimonials and Experiences
of Carnivores

- **Jurriaan** is 32 years old from the Netherlands. He is a Health Coach and personal trainer, and he has a story about his journey in search of the perfect and healthy diet. In his words, "I started a plant-based diet. In the beginning it felt really good but that was just for a couple of months. Pretty soon after starting this diet I got into trouble.... After two years on a plant-based diet I was burnt out." After lots of denials and questions as to why things were not working out for him, he had to look inwards to the problems and deficiencies of the plant-based diet and he came across vitamin B2 and Vitamin D deficiencies.

In a quest for a solution, Jurriaan went back to eating meat in small amounts and he began to feel better. The breakthrough for him was coming across Shawn

Baker at the Joe Rogan podcast. The rest they say is history. He has been on the carnivore diet ever since.

Jurriaan listed some benefits he has gotten from the carnivore diet so far and they are some of the benefits I have listed in earlier chapters

- Muscle gain

- Mental alertness (cure from depression, mood swings and mood swings)

- Correction of bipolar disorder

- Cure for inflammation

- Better health and digestion.

Jurriaan's advice to persons interested in the diet is that learning is key. "Learn about bioavailability; learn about human history. Try to understand why this diet can be good for you. Listen to your body, don't just blindly follow mainstream media, and choose for your health."

These are his final words in an interview conducted with the author of Ketogenic Endurance. "I got my life back. To be honest, I have been in a dark place for a long time, and some days I still can't believe that I have found the answer. Maybe this sounds crazy but I feel this way of eating has saved my life.

Another testimonial is from a 72-year-old Carnivore; this person had just completed 4 months on the Carnivore diet made up of beef, chicken, eggs, bacon, cheese, and fish. 4.25lbs was lost every month for four months but this is not the only testimonial in these few months. Others include:

- Improved mood

- Lower blood pressure

- Energy

- Bone strength

- Increased physical and mental strength

- Absence of hunger pains

- Cure for type 2 diabetes

These are the words of the 72 years old who currently feels 20: "…all of these benefits were from eliminating all fruit and vegetables. I look at vegans as people who are suicidal and they want to take as many other people with them. I don't know why this work but my guess is that the carnivore diet uses the nutrients more efficiently, but that's just my opinion."

A husband and wife have been on the carnivore diet for months, and their test results already testify of the goodness of the diet. Weight loss and strength are two major testimonies the couple has shared. Their meals are grass-fed beef, grass-fed butter, and omega 3 egg. They also eat burger patties without bun, with cheese and bacon twice a week to keep things interesting.

In the words of the wife, "my hubby's back pain is gone, sleeps without waking up at night, we both have more energy since we started this diet and we have lost weight. Overall, carnivore diet is working for us".

An experimental carnivore has also expressed her enthusiasm, as well as her findings so far. Currently, on fasting, she has high hopes for the carnivore diet. According to her, it has been three months and she already feels amazing on the carnivore diets. These are her words " I want this to be true because the foods that should be eaten are by far my favorite foods. I feel amazing on the carnivore diet."

Someone who has been a carnivore for quite a long while and has plans to be a carnivore for life also makes a comparison between the carnivore diets and other diets out there. According to this person, "personally I have zero interest in what other people eat. I'll eat carnivore likely for the rest of my life but if others are happy eating all plants or omnivore, as long as they are healthy and happy, good for them"

A carnivore for over one year also experienced a major change in terms of health issues. According to this carnivore, observing the carnivore diet does not require you to bother much about how to get your nutrients because muscle meats provide practically all the nutrients you might need. These are the results of the diet "before I began eating the carnivore diet, my life was a mess as I was always dealing with some sort of health issue. But for the last 13 months, I have been on this diet and I feel amazing."

For some persons, autoimmune and depression issues are the benefits gotten from the carnivore diet. Another person who began the carnivore journey after hearing about Jordan Peterson and his daughter also experienced wonders from the diet after a year on the diet. 'For anyone who is on the fence, I highly recommend it' is the encouragement from this satisfied person.

There are many testimonies from members of the carnivore diet worldwide, and you can get hold of more testimonies and get connected to other persons who have been on the diet and have been reaping the health benefits from the diet.

Like I said earlier, the testimonies you get depends on who you ask, but everyone has a story or two to tell that will show you that the benefits of being a carnivore are not just in word alone but people are living the benefits and will continue to live it in time to come.

Downsides Of The Carnivore Diet?

There is nothing infinitely perfect, and while I can choose to tell you that everything is smooth, perfect and totally without risk, there are some things that are worth considering as far as this diet is concerned.

- May not be suitable for some population

The carnivore diet is not ideal for everyone, although we would look into it in more detail in successive chapters. Persons who react to protein cannot afford to be on this diet.

Also, some persons like pregnant mothers, newborns and children are on special nutrients and so they cannot be on this diet.

- Deficiency of some diets: according to a dietician at the Ohio State University Wexner Medical Center in Columbus, RD, Liz Weinandy, like every other diet, there are downsides of the carnivore diets. According to her, when you completely cut out one food group there are bound to be deficiencies and effects as a result. This is why we have the steps you go through when switching the carnivore diet; these foods are removed slowly and in stages so that the body can recover and get used to the new food.

Also, some persons occasionally take vegetables and other kinds of foods if they think it is necessary to do so. Regardless, some persons have lived and are living solely on the carnivore diet and they are healthy and well.

- One a general note, it will take a lot of effort and will power actually to start and go through this diet but as I have often stated, it would be very rewarding in the end. Some challenges you would face include getting rid of your very best meals and habits and just like you would emotionally react to this change, your body would respond too.

But we know that nothing good comes easy so regardless of the challenges you might face, in the end, it is all geared towards a better, smarter and healthier you.

From the medical angle, we have not had many researches, and clinical trials carried out on the carnivore diet. Most of the claims and complaints that have been raised against the diet often come from a place of sheer resistance by persons especially vegans who are pretty set in their ways and feel like anything else other than their way of life or diet is wrong and unacceptable.

Regardless of all this, before you start on this diet ensure you properly understand your body and health; see a physician if possible to be sure that you can embark on this journey without any particular harm to your health for one reason or the other.

In the next chapter, we would be looking at the best ways to optimize your carnivore diet for better wellbeing and bountiful effects on your mind and body. Stick close as we continue on this journey to what might probably the most beneficial and effective diet you have ever gone on.

Chapter Eight: Best Ways To Optimize A Carnivore Diet

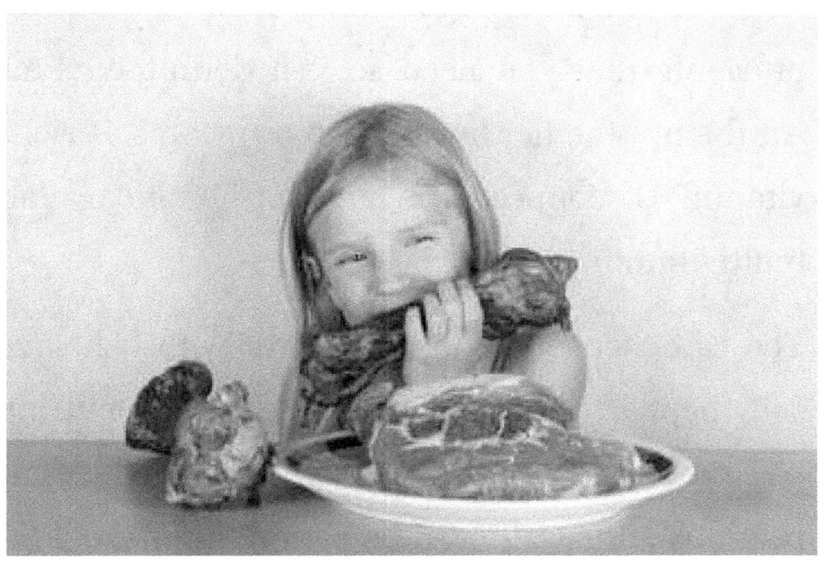

When you get started on a carnivore diet, you are taking your body a whole 360 degrees to another angle that you are not used to, and this change might happen really smoothly for some, but come with some difficulties and challenges for others.

Here are a few ways to optimize a carnivore diet and get lots of nutrients that people claim cannot be gotten from animal-based foods.

1. Eat Liver

Liver is a part of animal flesh and so it constitutes something you can eat without being said to have fallen off the bandwagon. Liver is filled with many nutrients that you need so you definitely should eat them. Whether liver of fish or meat, it is rich in vitamin D, copper, iron and lots of bioavailable multivitamin.

You can choose to cook your liver with fish sauce, salt, pepper, and little oil to get you a nutrient-packed meal, or get frozen liver tabs diced in small portions and swallowed or better still make a liver smoothie. Some persons blend raw liver and drink it, and yes, it might taste gross but it has been said to have cured iron deficiencies for some.

2. Eat Eggs

Some carnivores choose to restrict themselves to only meat and fish, but like I mentioned when giving the list of foods you can eat, you are also allowed to eat eggs as they are animal-based foods even though they are not quite the whole animal.

They also bring nutrients and benefits to the table so be sure to add them to your menu.

3. Eat lots of seafood

Vitamin D, omega 3, selenium, iodine, iron, copper and magnesium are few of the nutrients you can get from indulging in seafood. Get your hands on some salmon, oysters, mussels and other healthy seafood you can lay your hands on and trust me, you are bound to find some nutrients there that are not easy to come by.

4. Fast intermittently

A constant intake of muscle meat is perfect for muscle growth and general body health and well-being, but it is also important to fast intermittently to balance up the large amount of protein being sent into your body on a daily basis. And don't forget, the carnivore diet does not encourage too much of eating so taking a pause sometimes is advised.

5. Eat Quality meat and Animal based foods

Just eating meat is not enough; eating good meat is.. Processed meat is unhealthy and should be avoided

Grass-fed animals are the best sources of quality meat because they contain the original nutrients as taken in and digested by the animal. Organic meats are also pretty ideal, but it is important to ensure that you are having the best and healthiest meat that you can, because you might not get the results you are working towards if your carnivore diet in itself isn't healthy.

Getting confused? Not to worry, we will look into carnivore recipes and diet plans later so you will have an idea of what quality of meals you should be eating.

Chapter Nine:
How to Eat Cheap on the Carnivore Diet

GROUND MEATS	USDA REF NO	WATER	CALORIES	PROTEIN	TOTAL FAT	SATURATED FAT	MONO FAT	POLY FAT	CHOLESTEROL
TURKEY	05305	71.97	149	17.46	8.26	2.250	3.100	2.000	79
CHICKEN	05332	73.24	143	17.44	8.10	2.301	3.660	1.508	86
PORK 84% LEAN	10972	64.67	218	17.99	16.00	5.362	7.280	2.235	68
BEEF 90% LEAN	23562	69.50	176	20.00	10.00	4.058	4.353	0.344	65
BISON GRASS FED	17149	71.59	146	20.23	7.21	2.917	2.753	0.336	55

Comparing Ground Meats

Source: USDA National Nutrient Database For Standard Reference

Some persons fear that having to live on meat, fish and other animal-based food is more expensive than eating a regular diet that is a mash-up of everything. Some brows might have also been raised when I spoke about eating quality meat and one or two persons are already checking their purses to see if they can afford this diet but not to worry, there are a few ways to spend within your means as a carnivore and still get to eat the things you are supposed to.

- Buy what is on sale

Often, on a weekly or bi-weekly basis, supermarkets put things on sale, and they advertise them so you know what is sold at a cheaper rate at that time. You can look out for the best deals on offer by various supermarkets around you and choose the most affordable ones. For your steak, you can get healthy ground beef on sale and stock up the quantity you would need for a few days or a week. Apart from beef, you can also get other types of meat relatively cheaper than the price of beef, especially pork.

You can also get parts of chicken pretty cheap, like the drumsticks and the thighs so you can afford to get little of beef, chicken, and lots of pork. So whenever meat is on sale, run in with your shopping cart and stock up your fridge with cheap healthy meat.

- Take a break from steak if you can't afford it.

Who doesn't love their steak? Well, except for vegans of course. You might love to eat steak most of the time, but you might be unable to afford it as frequently as you need it. What then can you do?

There are two options available to you at this point; buy cheaper beef cuts that you nearly pass for the quality rib-eye steak you so much crave for. You can get sirloin steaks, beef short ribs, and top round steaks at relatively cheaper rates so that you don't have to go off your steak diet totally and also don't spend all of your money.

The second option is to take a break and go on a no-beef diet for a while, at least until you can afford to shop in those quarters again. While you are off beef, make your meals of pork, fish, chicken, and eggs for the time being; get variety of meals out of the kind of meat you can afford and believe me, you won't be missing beef for a while; at least not until you get enough money to get back into the supermarket for some beef.

- Buy directly from the butcher

Supermarket deals are pretty cool, but buying straight from the farmer or butcher who supplies the supermarkets is way cooler, and cheaper too.

Buying from the butcher can get you the best and freshest meat parts at nearly half the price you would get them at the supermarket. Remember how I spoke about grass-fed and finished beef? What better place to get them than from the local butcher in your town?

You can try connecting with a local butcher and agree on buying the parts of meat you need in bulk and believe me, it will come with lots of discounts, and you have your meat packed in the fridge just where you need them.

- Keep the eggs very present.

Eggs are special in many ways; they are very nutritional, they are extremely cheap, and they can be prepared in a thousand and one ways.

Anytime you want to go on a tighter budget, or even just for the fun of it, get into eggs quite a bit and you would find that you can make so many different sumptuous meals out of eggs even as you get the protein, fat, and cholesterol it has to offer you.

There are a thousand and one ways to make your eggs every day: scrambled, boiled, fried, grilled, waffled, or it can be deep-fried. Get into the internet and you will find out that you have been stuck to one or two basic methods when you have a plethora to choose from.

Don't be afraid to get the eggs in, even if you wish to do that every day.

Chapter Ten:
Can You Do This?

If you recall, when I talked about the downsides of the carnivore diet in chapter 7 I mentioned that not everyone can practice the carnivore diet. Even among those who can practice, there are different levels to which some persons take theirs.

We will be answering this important question now and finding out who can live on the carnivore diet and who cannot.

Who is the carnivore diet good for?

- Those looking for a change of diet, lifestyle and looking to cut out unhealthy meals and eating habits

- Persons with autoimmune diseases. The carnivore diet has shown amazing results when it comes to the management and treatment of this disease so people take up this diet to correct this health problem.

- Those who have tried keto and other low carb diets without getting their expected results.

- For persons suffering from food intolerance, going on the carnivore diet will help eliminate every other food item and then assist in finding out what food agrees with their system and what food doesn't

- Persons looking to lose weight reset their taste buds and rejuvenate their metabolism.

Who should not go on the carnivore diet?

As amazing and highly rewarding this diet is, some persons cannot afford to be part of it because of a trait, health issue or condition.

- Individuals who are prone to food and eating disorders should not try this diet; in fact, they shouldn't go on any form of diet at all, and this is totally for their own sake.

- Those who have chronic diseases and extreme health conditions might have to check with their doctors first to confirm if they can handle such extreme diets even with their illnesses.

- Persons suffering from chronic kidney diseases should not follow this diet; this is because they need to greatly limit their protein intake, and all the meals in this diet are majorly protein-based.

- Cholesterol sensitive people might have to be careful about this diet to avoid consuming too much cholesterol which they might react negatively to.

- Pregnant women are also advised not to eat the carnivore diet. The reason for this is not because the diet is harmful but because pregnancies have their peculiarities and there has not been much research done concerning the carnivore diet and pregnancy

Chapter Eleven:
What Kind Of Carnivore Are You?

While introducing this book, I explained that some carnivores take up extreme diets and food patters while some are not so extreme. A couple of carnivores allow cheese and milk in their diets while some do not. Some other carnivores take a break once in a few weeks to eat vegetables or treat themselves to a snack before going back to their diet. And a few others design their meals specially to suit their needs and preferences.

There is a general classification of carnivores into three kinds of categories, although there are so many persons practicing different unique types of this diet. Let's take a look at the major three

- **Hardcore Carnivore**: persons with incredible discipline who can go through with this diet. Those who crave meat and can definitely live on meat only as well as those you have tried keto before and are willing to go even further for the sake of their health are hardcore carnivores or likely to be.

- **Everyday Carnivores**: those who love meals like meat, scrambled eggs and cheese, steak, fish and other animal-based plants but cannot let go of some things like coffee and butter are likely everyday carnivores; they are almost hardcore but make a few compromises based on their preferences.

- **Weekday Only Carnivore**: people in this category take breaks often from their carnivore lifestyle, especially on weekends when they have outings, attend social gatherings or spend time with family. They do not want their personal diet to affect their relationships with other people so they take breaks. Some others just choose the weekends to take breaks and eat a few fruits and vegetables as a treat or present to themselves after a week of sticking to the carnivore diet.

Whatever category or class you fall into does not matter, what matters is ensuring you are taking it seriously and consistently to reap all of the benefits associated with this diet. Some persons don't even fall into any category as they decide to tweak the diet whatever way they choose to.

In the end, your mental, physical and emotional health is what we are working on perfecting by indulging in this zero-carb, animal based diet plan so do whatever you choose to the best of your ability.

Chapter Twelve:
Some Carnivore Recipes

The thought of eating only animal-based food for even a month might seem really daunting, but it is possible and even easier to put together than you can imagine. There are many things you can do with your meat, fish and eggs that would keep it looking and tasting new every time you eat it.

The most short-sighted comment anyone can make would be saying that there is nothing to eat when it comes to carnivore diet. You might think that it would get boring and become a drag by eating the same thing, but this is very far from the truth.

There are so many things in the mix for a carnivore diet, so many meals you can whip up with your meat, fish, eggs, cheese and milk if you don't mind including that as well.

These foods have been loved and eaten by many carnivores and even the non-carnivores who love to have a good meal; I can assure you that your next favorite meal is currently on this list I am about to put out.

- **Italian Burgers**

This simple burger recipe is very common and adaptable and it fits into any eating plan you are on. All you need for this burger is grass-fed ground beef, garlic powder, Italian seasoning and onion powder.

You simply mix the meat with all of the seasoning, form patties out of the mixture, and cook it up. You can also give it a shallow fry or grill it and you're good to go.

As simple as the meal is, it is autoimmune compliant.

- **Bacon-Wrapped Salmon**

Made with bacon, olive oil, filets of salmon, tarragon, with lemon as an optional ingredient, this dish is class enough to make the menu of a five-star restaurant or party.

This meal is tasty, attractive, and also a very low carb dish. The bacon helps to cut through the fattiness of the fish and also enhances the sweetness.

- Fish Bone Broth

This is a healthy drink made with fish head, ginger, leek, water, lemon and salt. Hardcore carnivores might not be interested in this drink, but others might be open to taking it.

Rather than throwing away your fish head and garlic after cooking, you can make the drink and have it; it is very nutritious and can also be used as flavor when cooking meat.

- **Garlic Bacon-wrapped Chicken Bites**

This is one really classy meal, and it looks eye-catching too. You might pay a lot for them if they're on the menu of a restaurant but you can get it done by yourself using chicken breast, bacon and garlic powder.

It is easy to cook, gets done on time, and can be eaten by everyone everywhere; trust me; it has been served at many expensive parties.

- **Marinated Grilled Flank steak**

Who doesn't love some great steak?

This recipe uses many powder seasonings, but you can omit by choice. The major ingredients include flank steak, garlic, coconut oil, apple cider vinegar, ginger, onion, dried thyme, lemon.

After cooking the meat with the ingredients till its soft, grill till your taste.

- **Slow Cooker Bacon and Chicken**

Chicken breasts and bacon are the two major ingredients for this dish. You can also add dried thyme, olive oil, salt, and dried rosemary.

Shred the chicken and bacon first and add the ingredients of your choosing and the end result is simply amazing. You can eat it with lettuce if you are open to that or simply have it like that.

- **Slow Cooker Pork**

This pork recipe keeps it simple with just pork shoulder, salt and ginger powder. You can cook pork in bulk with this recipe and save some for later, especially when you are on a no-beef budget, or you only want to enjoy some days of pork meat.

- **Pan-Fried Pork Tenderloin**

This is another simple and nice pork recipe that requires a bit of caution to prevent overcooking. The best way to enjoy it is when the meat is soft and juicy but not overcooked. With this one, less is more in terms of cooking time and when you turn off you should leave the meat to rest for a while before eating.

- **Chicken Bacon Skewers**

A combination of chicken and bacon that is set to get your taste buds on fire with just a few extra seasonings like salt and garlic powder.

First thing you do is to chop the chicken into bits, roll the bacon and then place them on the skewers. You can also make use of an oven if you choose and your meal would be ready in no time.

- **Crispy Indian chicken drumstick**

This meal is quick to prepare using Indian drumstick, salt, garam masala, and coconut oil. Garam masala is a traditional Indian spice that adds seasoning and taste to the drumstick. Ensure the meat is dry before you add the seasoning so as to get the crispy result when it is done.

- **Grilled Chicken Drumsticks with Garlic Marinade**

Chicken drumsticks, garlic, olive oil, sea salt, garlic, and lemon juice is the ingredients for this one. The garlic adds taste and flavor to the grilled chicken as well as the lemon juice.

- **Crispy Oven Roasted Salmon**

For this one, you are left to choose which seasoning would go along with the salmon filet, coconut oil, and sea salt which are the basic ingredients. If you want to keep it simple then you can sprinkle with salt and send the fish into the oven.

- **Garlic and Herb Bison Roast**

This meal is a gluten-free recipe with grass fed-bison roast, garlic and olive oil as its major ingredients alongside thyme and sage which is optional.

- **BBQ Chicken Liver And Heart**

Highly nutritious and full of flavor, this organ meat recipe has chicken liver, hearts alongside sea salt as its basic recipe. After spicing and cooking, you place them in the sticks, grill them, and you are good to go.

There are many things to try with animal-based foods, some that have not even been discovered yet, so if you think it is hard to make meals out of fish, meat and eggs, then you just haven't opened your eyes to the world of carnivores yet.

There are many more recipes out there for you to research and try out as you start or continue your journey as a carnivore. Explore, and enjoy what you find.

Chapter Thirteen: Carnivore Diet Meal Plan

The start of your journey into the world of carnivores might be an exciting one, but on top of that, you would still need guidance especially as regards drawing up a meal plan.

It is time to ditch the generic meal plan you have been using all your life that makes you think it is okay to eat something that you definitely shouldn't eat. While I urge you to start up with a new carnivore meal plan, I am going to point you in the right direction as to the number of meal plans you can begin practicing spanning from a few days to a few months.

One-week Carnivore Diet Meal Plan

If you are about starting your first week and you wonder what your shopping list and food timetable should look like, here is a brief peek at a one week plan I recommend for you.

	DAY 1	DAY 2	DAY 3	DAY 4	DAY 5	DAY 6	DAY 7
LUNCH	Ground Beef 80\20	Roaste d Lamb chops	Roaste d Pork belly	Roaste d fatty fish with butter	Beef steak	Roaste d pork chops	Grilled meat organ
DINNER	Chuck Roast	Seared beef steak	Ground Beef 85\15	Slow cooked Beef steak	Hambu rger patties and bacon	Roaste d fatty fish with tallow	Crispy cooked chicken

The table above is not a set- in stone kind of guidance but just offers you some directions on how to go about making the meal plan; you can choose to add or take away something depending on your personal preference.

Although the template I have given does not give room for breakfast, a daily diet consisting of breakfast, lunch, and dinner can have breakfast started up with cooked, fried or baked eggs with the option of cheese. The reason breakfast is noticeably absent is that most persons prefer to skip breakfast or at least skip one meal in the day to keep it light.

How To Make It Through The First 30 Days Of The Carnivore Diet

Like I noted in when giving you the steps to becoming a carnivore, the early few days, weeks and as far as the first one month is often the hardest time because your system is going through something totally different from what you have been doing.

While it might be easy to draw up your meal plan for a few weeks or even a month based on what I have shown you, there are things you have to watch out for, understand and practice to make it easier on you.

- Don't be moved by the urge to quit

You are going to mourn and complain a lot, this I can assure you of. Whether it is because you miss your previous meals, or you are finding it hard sticking to just animal-based food, or your body is reacting to the change, you would have to hold on.

You are likely to have spells of headaches, fatigue, energy drop, and general body weakness; this is simply because your carb intake has suddenly dropped alongside other nutrients your body has gotten used to.

Rather than running for the hills, give your body time to adjust and get used to your new diet, and you will be fine in no time. Make out time to sleep, avoid engaging in too much work, rest a lot when you feel the need to.

- You might be unable to control your appetite for a while

Your appetite would be a mess for a while; some days you would want to eat everything that crosses your line of vision, but some other times you would not even have the slightest interest in anything. Suffice to say your appetite might face some major mood swing but you will adjust well before you know it.

In worst cases, you might have the intense desire to eat something outside the carnivore diet, but if you can overcome it, don't cheat. However, if you must cheat, try not to go for foods too far outside the carnivore diet list because it might be hard getting back. You can get something that falls close to the carnivore diet but would also sort your cravings so you can get back on track.

- Get a blood test done before you start and during the first few months

As much as you might expect miracles from this diet, you should not jump in blindly without ensuring that it is doing something good for you.

Before you start the diet, visit the hospital to get a blood test done and understand where you are health-wise and physically so that you can study and analyze changes that occur over time.

Ensure you take note of changes in energy level, weight, digestion and general body wellness. Don't forget that some persons are not supposed to be on this diet for one reason or the other and they might not reap the goodness of the diet if they try.

So pay proper attention to your body and health, ensure that the diet is getting you to a better place; only then should you continue.

- You might face bowel challenges

For many persons, the first few weeks into the diet, they face constipation mostly due to the absence of as much fiber as they used to consume before. Some other persons, however, suffer cases of diarrhea and in worst-case scenarios, it might last for as much as a week but according to a few carnivores who experienced this, it almost always sorts itself out.

According to Baker Shawn, diarrhea is pretty common but you should continue regardless and things would get better.

In these first 30 days and even after, you are likely going to face challenges along the way that you have a hard time understanding or solving; this is where reading, studying and getting in touch with others who have progressed far in this diet would help.

In the FAQ section, I will try as much as possible to answer questions about many cases that might not come up in these chapters but might be essential for you to as you move on.

Chapter Fourteen: Comparing and Contrasting Keto and the Carnivore Diet

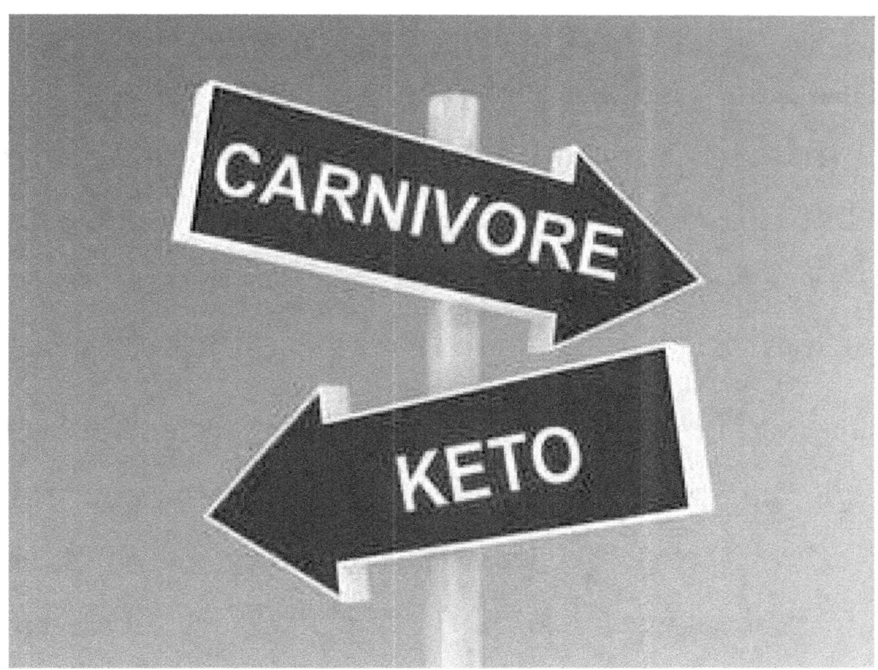

Carnivore diet and Ketogenic are probably the most compared and confused diets and the reasons for this are not far-fetched.

Carnivore diet and keto are pretty similar in a few ways, and people often try these diets for the same reason although the carnivore diet has been known to work faster and better. Regardless of their different unique nature, people often confuse, misunderstand and outright mix up both diets, so I am going to be drawing up major differences that set them apart just as I point out the similar traits they share.

The major reason people confuse keto and carnivore is that they are both aimed at cutting down carbs while increasing protein and fat-based nutrients. However, where keto stops, carnivore goes even farther.

The keto diet was originally tried and tested to treat epileptic patients although its uses now span past all of those areas, so when persons say there is no clinical backing for keto or even carnivore diet, I am forced to set the record straight with them. The major aim of this diet is to reduce carbs to the barest minimum, increase the consumption of fat and protein, which would result in the body-switching its energy source to dietary fat thereby leading to healthy weight loss.

The Carnivore diet, like I have pointed out in earlier chapters, has its main aim as eliminating plant-based and high carb foods while sticking to only animal-based food except for a few dairy products.

Let's take a quick look at some major differences between both diets.

Differences Between Keto and Carnivore Diets

1. The Carb allowance vs. disallowance

When you are on a ketogenic diet, you are allowed a little amount of carbs in your meals, and this falls around 50 grams or less daily. This is more flexible than the carnivore diet and also allows you to satisfy some food cravings that would plague you from time to time.

Keto also offers you the freedom to add vegetables to your protein meals giving you something to work with when trying to diversify your meals.

The carnivore diet is not as flexible as keto in terms of allowing carbs, fruits, and even fiber; for carnivores, they should be kept off the menu totally if possible.

2. Frequency of meals

Carnivore diets often limit food intake to thrice or even twice a day, alongside fasting periods that could also extend the time you get to eat.

When on a keto diet, however, food intake is spread through as much as five times a day while calculating the number of caloric intake that goes with each meal. Once again, carnivore is stricter than keto in this regard.

3. Handling cravings

The allowance of vegetables and other sources of fiber in keto food make it easy to survive cravings because you can get a taste of that thing you crave. While carnivore diet will not allow you to give in to cravings too often except by personal decision, it builds your self-control and saves you from wanting to run after some snack or drink anytime the feeling arises.

4. The ration of Macronutrients obtainable

Ketogenic diet keeps the ratio of carbs at 10% while having fat at 60% and protein at 30%; this keeps the production of healthy fat coming from calories and protein.

For carnivores, however, the risk of keeping the carbs present is not worth it especially when compared to its benefits so it is better to get all the nutrients needed from protein and fat and avoid carbs as much as we possibly can.

5. Low carb vs. zero carb:

Keto diets focus on keeping carb intake low through low carb vegetables and plants but the carnivore diet focuses on keeping all of the carb outside the door and putting a key in the lock.

In simple words, the differences between these two diets can be summarized with the fact both carnivore and keto alike allow consumption of fat and protein while aiming at taking off carbs from the diet, but while keto stops at putting prohibitive measures in place, the carnivore diet is stricter and more restrictive.

Similarities Between The Carnivore Diet And Keto

1. Weight loss

Both diets achieve weight loss because they both focus on cutting down calories however, the carnivore diet has been seen to offer faster and long-lasting results in this area most probably owing to its strict nature.

2. Increased energy levels

One benefit you can derive from practicing any of these diets is an increased level of mental and physical energy. Both diets ensure that you always have energy readily available for any form of work and you do not have to depend on some external energy booster or supplement.

3. The focus is on Healthy Fat

While other diets shun fat, keto and carnivore diet embrace healthy fat and work towards getting as much fat as possible into the body as it provides the fuel used to run the body.

Using fat as a source of energy not only ensures better mental and physical well-being, it also improves the level of alertness and agility of the body.

4. Spices and plant-based fats for nutritional value

As much as both diets focus on protein and fat, they also allow spices, fat is gotten from plant-based sources as well as seasonings in the preparation of their meals. For example, olive and coconut oil, apple cider vinegar, coffee and tea, salt and other spices.

Summarily, keto and carnivore diets are loved and adhered to because of the health benefits they offer as a result of taking out rather unnecessary food classes from your diet; but where keto stops in terms of results, effects and long term satisfaction, carnivore diet continues to provide quick and lasting solutions to large number of health challenges as we have seen in the unending testimonies of people who have lived on the carnivore diet or even switched from keto to carnivore because of surer and longer lasting benefits.

Chapter Fifteen:
Frequently Asked Questions About The Carnivore Diet

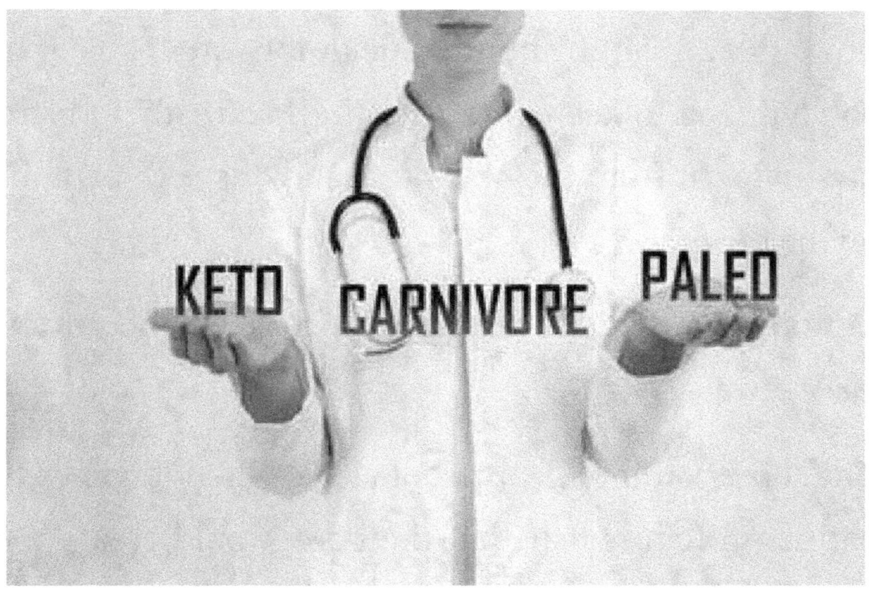

There have been many questions asked regarding the carnivore diet both by people looking to get into the diet as well as those who are already in but need someone to answer their questions and clear their doubts.

In this chapter, I will also address some statements posed by those who oppose the carnivore diet and let you know why their opinions do not matter.

You are probably going to have some of the theories you have believed all your life being debunked right now and it might be quite difficult for you to take it in so you need to keep an open mind, be ready to learn and unlearn from the questions and answers I will be laying down.

Question 1: Is there such a thing as too much protein?

The most common fear people have when it comes to eating protein is fear that the body would create too much glucose out of it, thereby increasing the blood sugar and insulin level. However, research has shown that this is not always the case.

Results from research in this area has shown that a rise in insulin is about 70% higher among persons who eat the standard diet high in sugar, starch, and carbohydrates than among persons who are practicing the low carb or zero carb lifestyle.

Testimonies from some persons have even shown that the carnivore diet helped cure their diabetes-related issues.

So you see, rather than being scared of protein when it comes to blood sugar level, you should be scared of everything but protein.

Question 2: Does it make sense to ditch vegetables?

Yes, it makes a whole lot of sense, and here is why.

You might think that we need them for their minerals, vitamins, and fiber but we can very much do without them, especially as they also stand the chance of putting us at health risks.

Many vegetables out there are high in starch; way too much starch that we could ever need. Fruits are also high in sugar.

On a general level, vegetables and other plants put people at risk of oxalates, phytates, antinutrients, and other unpleasant health situations.

Although the carnivore diet does not allow fruits and vegetables (especially at the beginning of your diet), you can choose to look out for the most healthy vegetables and fruits and add them sparingly from time to time, based on personal preference.

Question 3: How am I supposed to survive without Fiber?

We have been told right from time that fiber is an absolute necessity when it comes to digestion and helping food and waste pass through our guts and that without fiber, we would face major cases of constipation. **But here is the fact:**

The fiber you eat which is supposed to help your bowel isn't digestible in itself and just passes through: so what could be the use of that?

According to World Journal of Gastroenterology (2012), reducing or stopping the intake of fiber goes a long way to reduce constipation and other related bowel issues. Isn't that just something to be wowed about?

Author of 'From Fiber to the microbiome: low carb gut health' Dr. Paul Mason has also commented that persons who eat zero fiber meals are very regular with their bathroom visits and have no problems connecting to constipation.

What this tells you is that you can totally do without fiber, and you definitely should.

Source: Dr. Paul Mason

Question 4: Can I add dairy products to my carnivore diet?

The answer to this lies mainly in personal preference and level of strictness of the person going on the diet. Like we earlier clarified, some persons can choose to tweak the diet to suit their style while working with the general carnivore guidelines.

For some persons, allowing milk, cheese and the likes helps them to have variety in their meals and also makes it more enjoyable for them to practice the diet. For others, the lactose to be found within these dairy products is something they don't want to be present in their meals.

Overall, it depends on what you want to do, the reasons behind your actions and how much it would affect your overall health.

Question 5: Are spices allowed?

Well, more often than not, the major seasonings advisable for use are salt and pepper so as to keep it simple.

However, other spices are allowed to be used for creative different tastes and flavors although they should be kept at a minimum as well. How healthy are these spices? Is one question you should ask yourself every time you want to add them.

Question 6: Does the carnivore diet go well with exercise?

I have heard some persons wonder how they would be able to factor in exercises especially if they are always going to be 'very tired'. First of all, you will not always be tired; you would go through that for the first few days when your body is adapting but after that, you would be even stronger and more energized.

This is also where the importance of following every step towards becoming a carnivore comes in; if you start cutting out the vegetables, carbs, and oils slowly, your body would have already adapted to a large extent so it is not going to be too much of a change. In a few weeks, you are ready to exercise and work out as much as you want.

Question 7: Won't I suffer nutrient deficiencies?

It is very unlikely that you would suffer any deficiencies- if you are eating it right.

Red meat and fish contain a wide range of nutrients your body needs to work, including the not so common ones like Omega 3. Vitamins B6, B12, D, iron, zinc, protein, selenium and so much more nutrients are based on the foods that fall into the carnivore diet so you have nothing to worry about when it comes to available nutrients.

If there is something that cannot be found in the carnivore diet, it is most likely because you don't need it.

Question 8: Can I eat processed meats?

Meats are good for you, but processed meats, not so much. They are like the artificial and unhealthy version of meat, and they contain ingredients that are potentially harmful to your health.

Some researchers have also drawn a link between processed meats and some major health conditions, so it is a no for us.

Grass-fed animals are the healthier and wiser choice and that is what you should consume.

Question 9: How long would it take before I am totally adapted?

30 days is the usual adaptation period we have often had and observed and that is why the 30-day carnivore diet is quite a popular one.

What happens in this time frame is that your body is learning new ways to work that are different from what it has known all your life. Your system will get used to the absence of the grains and legumes with all of the carbs and then begin to make use of the fats and protein as an energy source to run with.

At the month's end, you should have totally adapted to the carnivore diet.

Question 10: Isn't all of this fat and cholesterol a recipe for heart attack?

There has been a widespread of misinformation about fats and cholesterol especially as it concerns heart health and the carnivore diet. Some persons think that once you consume anything high in fat you have put a gun to your heart ready to fire.

However, cholesterol is necessary for some very major functions in our bodies, without which we might be heading towards a health disaster. Take the brain, for example, it actually needs quite a high level of cholesterol to function and it takes about 25% of cholesterol residual in the body to put into good use with regards to thinking, learning, brain function, movement and even retention. Without the brain getting enough cholesterol, one would actually be at risk of memory loss, dementia, depression and even Parkinson's disease.

Low cholesterol has also been linked to the risk of nerve damages and also a cause of high death rates among the older population.

That is not all; cholesterol is a repair mechanism that becomes very important as we age. The cholesterol gotten from meat-based foods also promotes the repair of demyelinated lesions in the brain without which one would be at risk of dementia.

There are quite a number of dangers associated with low cholesterol; they include increased risk of cancer, risk of Alzheimer's disease, poor cognition, increased risk of stroke,, and even heart attacks.

So you see, cholesterol is not the bad guy he has been painted to be; the cholesterol gotten from animal-based plants is healthy, effective and offers you lots of health benefits like repairs of brain lesions, reduced risk of breast cancer, reduces mortality rate as well as colorectal cancer.

The next time someone tells you that high cholesterol results in heart disease, tell them that they are being short-sighted and painting cholesterol as the bad guy when they should probably be looking somewhere else.

Question 10: What about vitamin C, Don't I need it?

This is a major worry people have had, and it is not unfounded especially as we have heard statements on what the absence of Vitamin C can cause.

Generally, vitamin C has been described as the cure of virtually every disease and ailment out there just as the absence has been linked to the outbreak of Scurvy alongside fatigue, gum disease, potential death, bleeding, poor wound healing, and the likes.

But here's the thing; so far, so food in the past years, all of the persons who have gone on the carnivore diet have never had any issue of vitamin c deficiency and they were also not taking any supplements as well. So, how did they survive? You might ask.

Here is the thing, animals can make vitamin C by themselves internally and as a result, it is contained in their flesh. So, when you eat meat and fat alone, you can and will get vitamin c from the cooked meat.

Still having doubts? Let us go through the results of research conducted in this regard.

An anthropologist, Vilhjalmur Stefansson, made a decision to study the Inuit people of Alaska who are widely known to consume about 90% of meat and fish alone. Perhaps, he wanted to find out how come they didn't seem to be malnourished or suffering from any deficiency, or maybe he was just curious. Regardless, he visited Alaska and lived with these people.

Stefansson lived with the Inuit people for 9 years, and he joined their custom of eating only meat and fish for 6 to 9 months every year; he did this for 9 whole years but you know what? He did not suffer any health challenge for all of these years until he returned home.

While he was outwardly fine, there were doubts as to whether something might have gone wrong inside of his body so he moved to do a medical examination on himself. He moved to the Bellevue hospital in New York where he continued to eat nothing but meat and fat for 12 months. His meals were closely monitored all through this process, and by the end of the year, all of the food he ate was studied and a test was carried out on him to find out how he had fared.

Strangely enough, Stefansson had zero deficiencies, and he was in perfect health condition. Surprise!

This was a major finding, and it was published in 1930 by the Journal of Biological chemistry. Trust me; this is not the only study that has found people to be in a perfect state of health after being on the carnivore diet for long periods.

Simply put, you have nothing to worry about even in this regard; the carnivore diet contains all of the minerals and vitamins that you truly need.

Question 11: I Thought fruits were great for my health. What is going on?

Every one of us grew up hearing that fruits and vegetables are two things we should never go without because they are heaven and earth of good health and they had all of the fiber and antioxidants in the world that would keep us in perfect shape?

If you still believe this, you should pay attention to the facts in the next few sentences, according to Kevin Stock, author of *Your Drum*, a hardcore carnivore and self- experimental researcher.

- First of all, Fruit produces fructose rather than glucose as its sugar. And the thing with fructose is that it does not stimulate leptin, which lets us know when you are full so what it does to you is that it keeps you eating and filling up even when you should have stopped.

- Secondly, fruit has gotten more and more unnatural just as agriculture develops and modern food changes. So would you continue eating something that you probably shouldn't eat?

- People are getting impatient and no longer wait for fruits to get ripe on their own but pick fruits up from trees when they are unripe. They then treat the fruits with chemicals to ripen them quickly just so they can sell them to you.

As if this is not enough harm being done, the fruit itself when unripe have a very high toxic load as well as a protective hull to keep the predators away. So you have chemicals from the fruits and artificial chemicals all in one fruit you are eating to stay healthy.

Still want to eat fruits? That is highly doubtful.

Question 12: Won't I get fat from all of this fat?

No, you won't, and here is why.

In the absence of carbs and sugar and all of the things you are cutting out of your diet, your body is doing all the work it has to do with the protein and fat you have consumed. This fat then becomes the primary sauce of energy and the body uses a large amount of the fat you consume to run your internal processes.

So, in the end, you don't have the excessive fat you are scared of adding to your weight. The funny thing is, it is when you are on your standard diet consuming all of the snacks, drinks and foods you used to eat that you have to worry about getting fat.

So many questions have been asked about the carnivore diet, and people will continue to have questions as the knowledge of this diet continues to spread. I hope I have been able to help clear your doubts to a large extent and show you just what is in store for you when you become a carnivore. Now, let's wrap things up.

Conclusion:
Now you know, what happens next?

It has been quite a journey up until this point, and I hope it has been exciting and engaging for you as it has been for me.

We have gone through the history of the carnivore diet and where it stands alongside human history. We have also been able to get an assurance of the fact that an animal-based diet is so much healthier than you would ever think or imagine.

If the research and facts were not enough to build your conviction, testimonies and reports from persons who have lived and are currently living this lifestyle should.

The carnivore meal plan is also there to help you work through your first few days, weeks, and months on the diet.

We have also been able to debunk a few myths that have continued over the years as it concerns the carnivore diet and its hidden benefits.

At this point, I believe the next thing to do is to get started on this diet as soon as you can. Once you complete your first 30 days, you would literally be itching to go all the way.

There are a large number of people belonging to the carnivore communities on Facebook, Instagram, and other media platforms and probably even in your local communities. Connect with people, seek advice and directives from persons currently undergoing the diet and they would prove to be just the support group that you need on this journey.

Don't forget to make sure you actually can embark on this diet because, like we stated, some health conditions would make it difficult to reap the benefits of going on this diet.

All of the cures and benefits we have seen connected to this diet are bound to become a reality if you can actually go through with this diet.

I look forward to hearing from you, getting your testimonies, and helping you along in any way that I can.

You deserve perfect health, the perfect body, and the perfect life and I welcome you to that perfect life right now.